Steel and Stamina: Sculpting Strength for Men

Stephen N. Arnold

TABLE CONTENT

CHAPTER 1: ANATOMY AND FUNCTION OF THE MUSCLES

- Summary of the Muscular System
- Muscle Tissue Types
- Types of Muscle Fibers and How They Affect Strength
- The Neuromuscular Junction: Contraction through Communication
- The Fundamentals of Hypertrophic Muscle

CHAPTER 2: DIETARY TECHNIQUES FOR INCREASING MUSCLE MASS

- The Functions of Macronutrients in Bodybuilding
- Timing Nutrients to Optimize Muscle Synthesis
- Enhancement for Maximum Efficiency
- Nutritional Strategy for Building Muscle
- Hydration and Its Essential Function for Muscle Growth

CHAPTER 3: RESISTANCE TRAINING FUNDAMENTALS

- Resistance Training: Definitions and Uses
- Getting to Know the Equipment: From Dumbbells to Machines
- Form and Technique: Optimizing Performance, Reducing Damage
- Fundamentals of Programming for Novices
- The Principle of Progressive Overload

CHAPTER 4: COMPLEX EXERCISE METHODS

- Periodization: A Sophisticated Approach to Planning

- Explosive Growth Plyometric
- Movements of Isolation vs Compounds
- Unconventional Exercise for Increasing Strength
- Burnouts, Super Sets, and Drop Sets

CHAPTER 5: RECUPERATION TECHNIQUES
- The Value of Recuperation and Rest
- Sleep: The Unappreciated Source of Strength
- Active Rehabilitation: Methods and Advantages
- Overtraining Syndrome: Identifying and Avoiding It
- Mobility and Stretching Exercises

CHAPTER 6: CREATING THE PERFECT EXERCISE PROGRAM
- Making Reasonable Objectives
- Split routines versus full-body workouts
- Example Exercise Schedules for Different Fitness Levels
- Adapting Your Exercise to Your Development
- When and How to Adjust Your Daily Schedule

CHAPTER 7: STABILITY AND CORE STRENGTH
- The Function of the Core in Strength
- Exercises to Strengthen the Core
- Training in Stability to Prevent Injuries
- Including Core Tasks in Your Daily Routine
- Complex Core Exercises for Optimal Strength

Chapter 8: Olympic lifting and Powerlifting
- Overview of Powerlifting
- Olympic Lifting: An Overview of the Technology
- Principles and Practices of Power Training
- Including Strength Training Exercises in a Bodybuilding Program
- Safety and Equipment for Heavy Lifting

Chapter 9: Bodybuilders' Cardiovascular Exercise Program

MOTIVATION

"The body is not the source of one's strength.

The source is the human will."

In the midst of heavy lifting
and the whiff of resolve, it's important to keep in mind that
true strength comes from inside and is not contingent on
external factors. You push yourself past previous limitations
with every repetition, every set, and every day that you
return to the forge that sculpts your own essence.
This aphorism is a reminder that the actual substance being
tempered in the crucible of iron and sweat is not just
muscle, but the essence of your willpower.

CHAPTER 1

ANATOMY AND FUNCTION OF THE MUSCLES

Anatomy and Function of the Muscles Understanding the intricate architecture and the multifaceted functions of muscular systems serves as the cornerstone for comprehending how our bodies execute myriad tasks, ranging from the most mundane to the herculean. This comprehension not only enhances our awareness but also propels our efforts in muscle building.

- ## Summary of the Muscular System

The muscular system is an extensive network of tissues that facilitates movement, stability, and the power to manipulate our environment. Muscles are meticulously organized to maintain posture, generate heat, and provide the locomotive capabilities necessary for survival and interaction. This system is a marvel of biological engineering, with over 600 muscles working in harmony to orchestrate the symphony of physical actions that constitute human movement. Each muscle, from the minuscule in our inner ears to the majestic gluteus maximus, plays a pivotal role in our everyday existence. Their cooperative efforts afford us the ability to engage in activities as diverse as sprinting to catch a bus or finely tuning a musical instrument.

- ## <u>Muscle Tissue Types:</u>

Intriguingly, muscle tissue bifurcates into three distinct categories: skeletal, cardiac, and smooth muscles. Skeletal muscles, under voluntary control, are the workhorses driving our interactions with the physical world. Cardiac muscle, the tireless engine of our circulatory system, operates beyond the reach of our will, contracting ceaselessly to fuel our body with life-sustaining blood. Smooth muscle, found within the walls of organs such as the stomach and arteries, moves involuntarily, controlling the flow of substances within our bodies and maintaining essential functions without a moment's rest.

- ## <u>Types of Muscle Fibers and How They Affect Strength</u>
Delving into skeletal muscle reveals a tapestry woven from various muscle fibers. These fibers are classified into type I, type Ilia, and type Ibis, each with unique characteristics. Type I fibers, often referred to as slow-twitch fibers, are enduring powerhouses, allowing for prolonged activities such as distance running. Type II fibers, known as fast-twitch fibers, are recruited for their explosive power, essential in sprinting and weightlifting. The ratio of these fibers within an individual's muscles can predetermine their potential for strength and endurance, a testament to the genetic lottery each of us partakes in. However, through targeted training, one can sculpt their musculature to enhance the desired fiber type, pushing the boundaries of their innate capabilities.

8

- ## <u>The Neuromuscular Junction: Contraction through Communication</u>

The neuromuscular junction is a fascinating focal factor wherein frightened gadgets and muscular gadgets converge. It is right here that electrical signals from the mind are translated into the chemical messages that instigate muscle contractions. This process commences with a nerve impulse accomplishing the release of a motor neuron, freeing acetylcholine into the synaptic cleft. This neurotransmitter binds to receptors on the muscle fiber's floor, prompting a cascade of events leading to the sliding of actin and myosin filaments in the muscle cells—a technique culminating in contraction.

- ## <u>The Fundamentals of Hypertrophic Muscle</u>

Hypertrophy, the expansion of muscle fibers, is a complex version of resistance schooling. When muscular tissues are exerted past their accustomed depth, micro tears arise in the fibers. The next restoration technique, fueled by good enough nutrients and relaxation, fortifies the muscle tissue, making it larger and more potent than before. This adaptive reaction is the frame's foresight, preparing itself for future demands. It is a sluggish and painstaking procedure that requires constant exertion, nutrition, and healing. In short, the muscular device is a testimony to the complexity and adaptability of the human frame. With each stride, elevate, and stretch, our muscle tissues are in a perpetual state of flux, adapting to the stresses we impose upon them. Understanding the myriad functions and systems inside this gadget now not only fuels our appreciation but also guides our adventure closer to height and bodily shape. It is an adventure no longer for the faint of heart, but for those willing to learn, adapt, and persevere.

CHAPTER 2

DIETARY TECHNIQUES FOR INCREASING MUSCLE MASS

- **Macronutrients' Roles in Bodybuilding**
Proteins, carbs, and fats are macronutrients that can be vital to bodybuilding because they each have a wonderful effect on the development of muscle and standard physiological overall performance. Amino acid-based proteins are required for the synthesis of recent muscle fibers and for healing the micro tears due to severe resistance exercise. There is a widespread variety of protein resources to be had, starting from plant-based substitutes to whey isolates. Each has a completely unique amino acid profile, charge of absorption, and organic value; that's the proportion of protein absorbed from a given meal that is integrated into the proteins of an organism.

During excessive exercise, carbohydrates serve as the main electricity source and replace the glycogen reserves observed in muscles. High-GI carbs can speedily boost insulin and blood glucose levels, developing anabolic surroundings that are favorable for improvement. On the other hand, low-glycemic carbs offer an extended-lasting energy boost that is fine for sizeable exercise classes or for maintaining constant blood sugar levels all day.

Although they are regularly demonized in the weight loss plan enterprise, fats are really vital for plenty of organic features, which include the synthesis of hormones (in particular, increased hormone and testosterone, which might be crucial for the growth of muscle groups). Fish, nuts, and seeds include polyunsaturated and monounsaturated fats, which might be known to beautify cardiovascular health and can help with the absorption of fat-soluble nutrients, which are crucial for numerous organic tactic

- **Timing Nutrition to Promote Muscle Regrowth**

A well-planned nutritional timing technique can enhance muscle protein synthesis, which is critical for building muscle mass. Protein consumption soon after a workout may benefit from the "anabolic window," which is the time period for the accelerated state of muscle responsiveness to amino acids. This time range, which was previously assumed to be somewhat limited, ought to be virtually longer than formerly anticipated, presenting a greater enough window of opportunity for nutrient absorption. 2614

Consuming carbohydrates after working out can also speed up recovery by replenishing glycogen, especially when coupled with protein. Together, these two factors increase insulin production, which in turn helps muscle cells absorb glucose and amino acids. A well-planned daily carbohydrate intake that is in line with the body's circadian cycles and degree of physical activity guarantees maximum glycogen resupply and long-term energy.

- **<u>Improvement for Optimal Effectiveness</u>**
  Extra consumption can increase the effectiveness of a carefully thought-out diet. Through osmotic action and ATP resynthesize, creating monohydrate—which has been thoroughly researched and proven safe—increases muscle volume and power output. During calorie-restricted periods, branched-chain amino acids (BCAAs), namely leucine, valine, and isoleucine, may enhance muscle protein synthesis and reduce catabolism. Omega-3 fatty acids, which are mostly found in fish oil supplements, are hypothesized to improve the sensitivity of muscle protein synthesis to insulin and amino acids, hence offering a slight but significant benefit to muscle growth.

- **<u>A Dietary Approach to Muscle Building</u>**

  A comprehensive approach to nutrition is necessary for muscle amplification, matching macronutrient intake to the training load, metabolic rate, and recuperation requirements of the person. Gaining muscle frequently requires an excess of calories, but the increase must be carefully considered to prevent an excessive buildup of adipose tissue. The skill of fine-tuning a diet for muscular growth is based on an iterative process of calorie modification based on regular assessments of progress and body composition. As long as daily calorie and nutritional targets are reached, meal frequency and quantity can be adjusted to suit individual preferences, digestive comfort, and lifestyle factors.

- **<u>Hydration and Its Crucial Role in Muscle Building</u>**

Though often overlooked, hydration is the foundation of all elements of muscle metabolism. In addition to being a medium for dietary transit, water additionally performs a role in metabolic activities, which include the synthesis of adenosine triphosphate (ATP), which is vital for muscular contraction. Adequate fluid consumption is essential for the reason that dehydration can lower energy, accelerate fatigue, avoid muscle recovery, and hinder overall performance. Electrolytes, which include sodium, potassium, and magnesium, are crucial for nerve impulse transmission, muscle contractions, and fluid homeostasis. Consequently, ingesting meals or liquids high in electrolytes on a normal basis would possibly beautify rigorous workout applications and maximize muscle improvement.

This scholarly article provides an outline of the dietary approaches that can be important for gaining muscle tissue. It also discusses the capabilities of macronutrients in bodybuilding, the significance of timing vitamins, the possibilities of dietary supplements, a complete nutritional plan, and the need for hydration so that you can expand muscle. Because each aspect is complicated and shows a tapestry of organic relationships, individuals who need to broaden their muscle tissues through vitamins and schooling need to use a sophisticated method.

CHAPTER 3
RESISTANCE TRAINING FUNDAMENTALS

- ### Resistance Training: Meanings and Applications

Resistance schooling, which is once in a while pressured with electricity education, is an extensive category of sporting activities supposed to improve physical health through the application of external resistance to a muscle or muscle institution. One's very own body weight, resistance bands, weight machines, or unfastened weights can all offer this resistance. The most important targets are to boom bone density, boom muscular persistence, sell muscle hypertrophy, and increase total frame power.

Resistance training is used in many fields, from sports to rehabilitation, and it has several health benefits. It can increase metabolism, aid weight reduction, make the heart stronger, and promote intellectual wellness. Beyond the physiological, resistance education has an extensive effect on useful health, allowing people to perform day-to-day tasks more easily.

- ### Getting to Know the Tools: From Machines to Dumbbells

For newcomers, navigating the variety of resistance training equipment available might be intimidating. Dumbbells are versatile and need the stability of muscles during a workout. They have an extensive range of motion, which is essential for focusing on certain muscle groups and enhancing muscular balance.

Barbells are useful for complex exercises that work several muscular groups, such as squats and deadlifts, and they make it possible to lift larger weights. Resistance bands offer resistance during both the concentric and eccentric stages of an activity. They are portable and come in different tension levels. Weight machines are helpful for people who are recuperating from an injury or are not familiar with correct lifting methods because they provide a controlled environment and reduce the risk of harm by guiding the user along a predetermined course of movement.

- **<u>Form and Technique: Enhancing Efficiency, Minimizing Harm</u>**

One cannot stress the importance of form and technique enough. Using the right technique guarantees full muscle activation and lowers the risk of injury. It involves breathing patterns, regulated movement pace, and alignment of various body components. To avoid putting too much strain on tendons, ligaments, and joints, it is essential to learn proper technique before increasing weight or resistance levels.

To teach correct technique, coaches and fitness experts frequently use signals and hands-on assistance. As an example, they could suggest maintaining a neutral spine, placing the feet shoulder-width apart, or inhaling during the eccentric and exhaling during the concentric phases of movement. Every exercise has a distinct set of strategies that, when learned, greatly increase the safety and efficacy of training.

- ## The Foundations of Programming for Beginners

A beginner's resistance training program should be straightforward and concentrate on basic motions that build confidence and strength. All of the major muscle groups must be worked out during the programming, which should be done two or three times a week to allow for adequate recuperation.

A beginner's program could start with a full-body routine that consists of a lower-body exercise (like squats), a push movement (like a row), and a pull action (like a press). These fundamental workouts promote the balanced growth of the various muscular groups. Exercises can get more specialized as beginners progress, concentrating on certain muscles or movement patterns

- ## The Progressive Overload Theory

One of the essential thoughts of resistance education improvement is modern overload. It is critical for ongoing development and suggests the innovative elevation of strain carried out on the neurological and musculoskeletal structures. You can increase the weight you carry, boom the wide variety of repetitions or units, or change the quantity of time you relax in between units to obtain incremental overload.

Muscle fibers need to be pushed past their present limits, which allows you to broaden and adapt. This can also entail editing the workout routines to make them more challenging or varying the tempo at which they're achieved. It is essential to apply innovative overload cautiously and to check it closely to make sure that the increase is sustainable and does not have an effect on form or purpose.

"This chapter offers a basic overview of resistance training, including its description, applications, types of equipment available, the importance of correct form, basic program design for novices, and the fundamental idea of progressive overload. Every segment unites around the idea that mastering these fundamentals is the cornerstone of an effective and long-lasting strength training program. These basics serve as a benchmark for anyone just starting out on this route, guaranteeing a safe and efficient advancement".

CHAPTER 4
COMPLEX EXERCISE METHODS

- **Periodization: An Advanced Method of Scheduling**
Periodization is the methodical scheduling of physical or
athletic schooling. It entails gradually cycling through distinct
schooling program components over a certain amount of time.
It's a complicated technique that helps athletes and fitness
fanatics adjust their restoration, stay off plateaus, and reach
their height just in time for contests.

Using this technique, the training plan is divided into
numerous levels or blocks, each with a wonderful emphasis.
These levels include the macrocycle, which is the whole
schooling period, commonly lasting a year; monocycles,
which span a few weeks to numerous months; and
macrocycles, which generally last every week and involve

each day sports that might be specifically planned to improve the principle objectives.

A periodized plan typically starts with a phase of growing muscle, referred to as hypertrophy, and then actions into durations of power and energy, each of which, step by step, will increase in intensity while reducing in quantity. This machine permits the body to get better for the duration of much less extreme cycles, which no longer only improves performance but also reduces the chance of overtraining.

- ### **Rapid Development: Plyometric**

Plyometric workouts are designed to maximize muscular strength in the shortest amount of time. These exercises, which are also known as ploys or jump training, involve explosive movements like hops and leaps that instantly contract a muscle, utilizing the strength and suppleness of the surrounding connective tissues as well as the muscle itself.

Plyometric training improves muscular coordination, power (power is equal to strength times speed), and speed, which is useful for sports and other tasks requiring quick movements. Many sports, such as basketball, martial arts, and running, can benefit from this training.

- ### **Isolation vs. Compound Movements**

Leg extensions and bicep curls are examples of isolation exercises that focus on a particular muscle group and include movement around a single joint. By focusing on a single muscle, these motions enable people to increase muscular activation and maybe even hypertrophy.

Conversely, compound motions use several muscle groups and several joints during motion. Compound motions include exercises like bench presses, deadlifts, and squats. Because they imitate natural motions and demand more energy, these workouts are effective for increasing general strength and muscle development because they burn more calories and boost the hormone response, both of which are good for muscle building.

- **<u>Non-Traditional Strengthening Exercise</u>**
  In the quest for diverse and comprehensive strength development, unconventional training techniques are becoming more and more popular. Activities that offer the body a distinct challenge include kettlebell swings, Indian club training, and even strongman activities like tire flips and sled drags. These movements improve the body's connective tissues and joint stability, in addition to strengthening the muscles.

  These non-traditional techniques frequently combine elements of coordination, stability, and mobility, testing the body in three dimensions and giving rise to useful strength that can be used in sports and everyday activities.

- **<u>Drop sets, super sets, and burnouts</u>**

  Advanced schooling techniques, which include burnouts, high-quality sets, and drop units, aim to venture muscle mass past their comfort zones, cause muscular exhaustion, and promote hypertrophy. Burnout sets entail working out to bodily failure, or till the muscle is so tired that it is unable to do a repeat with the right form.

Super sets are when two sporting activities are executed again-to-again without a wreck in between. This can be carried out for opposed muscle groups to enhance workout depth and save time, or it can be completed for the identical muscle group to elevate depth.

Drop units are sporting activities where you work out till you reach your limit, then you definitely lower the load and keep going until you attain your restriction. This method lengthens the workout, draws in additional muscle fibers, and may provide a robust stimulus for muscular development. Through the usage of these advanced exercise techniques, human beings may also master superior strategies like periodization to organize their schooling, plyometric to improve explosive electricity, and the strategic use of isolation vs. compound sporting activities to maximize muscle increase. Incorporating non-conventional exercise techniques can also revitalize a schooling routine by providing new challenges for ongoing variation and development. Finally, through pushing the muscle into deeper states of exhaustion, intensifying strategies like burnouts, extraordinary sets, and drop sets can cause variations that cause expanded muscle hypertrophy and endurance. When used well, these state-of-the-art techniques preserve the key to unlocking unprecedented stages of performance and bodily power.

CHAPTER 5
RECUPERATION TECHNIQUES

- ### The Importance of Rest and Recovery

The foundation of every intense training program is recovery and rest. These are crucial times for the body to heal and strengthen, rather than just taking a break from exercise. Resting enough is essential for improving performance, preventing injuries, and maintaining general health. It gives the body enough time to rebuild damaged tissues, refuel, and adjust to the strains of exercise. Rest periods are just as important as exercises, since it's during these times that the body consolidates the improvements made from training.

- ### Sleep: The Underappreciated Power Source

Sleep is the only kind of rest and a critical thing for physical and intellectual healing, even though it is frequently neglected in a trendy, traumatic society. The development hormone, which is concerned with muscle development and restoration, is launched while you sleep. Sleep additionally gives the frightened system a time to unwind and regroup, which is important for maintaining the intellectual readability and muscular coordination required for education. Persistent sleep deprivation can prevent the outcomes of exercising, postpone recovery, cause hormone imbalances, and raise the chance of injury.

- **<u>Active Rehab: Approaches and Benefits</u>**

Active rehabilitation includes a variety of exercises intended to hasten the healing process following an accident and avert further harm. Active recovery, in contrast to passive rest, entails low-intensity exercise throughout the recuperation phase. By removing waste materials and increasing blood flow to the muscles, these exercises strengthen their structure without putting undue strain on them.

Examples of techniques include swimming, cycling at a leisurely speed, and mild running. Yoga and mild stretching are examples of active rehabilitation techniques that can help preserve mobility and lower the chance of muscular stiffness. This kind of recovery makes sure the body stays active, which facilitates a speedier and more complete return to optimal fitness.

- **<u>Recognizing and Preventing Overtraining Syndrome</u>**

When education quantity and depth surpass the frame's capacity for restoration, overtraining syndrome arises because of an imbalance between training and recuperation. Prolonged exhaustion, impaired features, emotional fluctuations, and heightened vulnerability to infections are some of the signs.

A nicely-deliberate schooling routine that contains enough relaxation and a healthy weight-reduction plan is necessary to save you from overtraining. Ensuring mental well-being, editing intensity, and preserving an eye on the education of the masses are important measures to prevent this dangerous situation. Long-term setbacks may be prevented, and schooling consistency may be preserved with the resource of early detection and management.

- **<u>Exercises for Mobility and Stretching</u>**

Exercises for flexibility and mobility are, on occasion, overlooked in the choice of extra-active exercises, but they're vital for maintaining functional range of movement and preventing injuries. Stretching goals to lengthen the muscle mass and tendons, while mobility sporting events goal the motion of joints, ensuring they can flow freely and painlessly.

By including these sporting activities in one's program, you can still improve performance, reduce the threat of muscular imbalances and accidents, and enhance posture. Before working out, dynamic stretching—which entails shifting body parts while step-by-step growing reach, pace, or both—may be very useful. Static stretching, on the other hand, is better for cooling down after exercising because it includes retaining a stretch for a while.

All matters considered, healing techniques are critical to the lengthy-term effectiveness of any physical training routine. They cover a huge variety of techniques, from the fundamental importance of sleep to the advantages of energetic rehabilitation and the requirement of mobility exercises. It is equally vital to understand overtraining syndrome and discover ways to prevent it for long-term performance and health. When used wisely, these healing strategies promote both mental and physical recovery, strengthening the frame's adaptability and potential for improvement.

CHAPTER 6
CREATING THE PERFECT EXERCISE PROGRAM

- **Creating Reasonable Goal**

Establishing attainable objectives is the first step in creating the ideal workout routine. As a kind of lighthouse, goals inspire motivation and direct the path. Reasonable goals take individual goals, lifestyle restrictions, and physical levels into account. They must be time-bound, relevant, measurable, achievable, and specific (SMART). It is more realistic, for instance, to set a goal of cutting two minutes off your 5K time in six months rather than trying to win a marathon with little to no running experience.

- **<u>Split Plans vs. Whole-Body Exercises</u>**

The preference between split exercises and full-frame physical games is primarily based on education degree, timetable, and private goals. Split routines provide for greater targeted schooling and sufficient healing time for each muscle institution by specializing in various muscle agencies on separate days. This technique is regularly chosen by those who can commit multiple days per week to education and who want to gain more muscular mass and strength.

On the other hand, complete-body sporting events involve operating out every major muscle organization in an unmarried session and are normally achieved twice or three times per week. This is a mainly useful technique for inexperienced people, time-constrained individuals, and those who want to shed pounds and enhance their health. Because of the improved total intensity of the exercise, it promotes balanced muscle growth and fat burning.

- **<u>Sample Workout Plans for Various Levels of Fitness</u>**

Beginners can begin with a basic, complete-frame exercise program that specializes in two to three fundamental activities like push-ups, rows, and squats. As they improve, they may transfer to a cut-up routine, focusing on wonderful body areas on numerous days. For instance, they could integrate the legs and biceps on the third day and the chest and triceps on the second one.

Intermediate exercisers should split their workouts into four days: two days for legs that also involve core work, and separate sessions for upper body push and pull activities. A five- or six-day split may be used by advanced fitness enthusiasts to further isolate specific muscular groups, such as the shoulders, arms, chest, back, and legs. One day might be set aside for accessory motions, and a second leg day could be used to target weak areas.

- **<u>Customizing Your Workout for Your Personal Growth</u>**

People's bodies change as they advance, leading to plateaus. As such, it's important to modify the training regimen on a frequent basis. Exercise modifications, weight increases, and changes to the rep range can all offer fresh challenges for ongoing improvement. To further push the body and promote growth, additional techniques like supersets, drop sets, or periodization can be included.

It's also essential to periodically reevaluate goals in order to match the fitness regimen with changing goals. For example, if the original objectives were to lose weight and they have been achieved, new objectives may be to build strength or define your muscles.

- **<u>When and How to Modify Your Everyday Routine</u>**

Changes in objectives, occasions, and activities in lifestyles all require adjusting one's workout routine. Adaptability is essential. To account for variations in strength ranges or time regulations, one must feel free to move sporting events to other instances of the day or week, regulate the depth of the activity, or shorten its length.

High-intensity C language training (HIIT) is a useful short-term solution for maintaining health when time is limited. If healing is a problem, it may be beneficial to add more rest days or deal with energetic recuperation through the use of low-depth sports like yoga or strolling.

Monitoring improvement on a normal basis the use of information and physical opinions can help determine whether or not to change the exercise. If there are regressions or stops within the software's development, it can be time to check it and make the vital modifications.

In the end, designing the proper exercise routine is a dynamic procedure that revolves around personalization. Establishing practical goals establishes the foundation, and choosing the right exercise breaks up prepared development. Sample schedules offer a framework that may be adjusted as fitness ranges change. Program momentum can be sustained by progressively modifying it, and application suitability for evolving lifestyles may be guaranteed via know-how and how to make adjustments to every day workouts. When those components are mastered, workout software that is comprehensive and efficient is created, which complements fitness and well-being for lifestyles.

CHAPTER 7
STABILITY AND CORE STRENGTH

- **The Role of the Core in Power**

The core is an essential component of almost all body motions, serving as the pivot between the upper and lower bodies. It consists of the muscles of the pelvis, lower back, and hips, in addition to the muscles of the abdomen. Maintaining good posture, guaranteeing effective energy transmission, and giving stability to the entire body all depend on having a strong core. A strong core improves overall strength capabilities by facilitating more control over movements and minimizing the strain on the spine.

- **<u>Core Strengthening Exercises</u>**

Exercises that focus on all the muscles in the central body segment will strengthen the core. Conventional workouts such as planks, crunches, and bridges are helpful. But including exercises that use several planes of motion might result in a more thorough development of the core. These comprise stability-testing activities like medicine ball tosses, lateral motions like side planks, and rotational workouts like Russian twists.

Stability aids like Swiss balls or suspension systems, which make the core muscles work harder to maintain balance, may be used in advanced core workouts. Furthermore, when done correctly, complex exercises like overhead presses, deadlifts, and squats are very efficient in activating the core muscles in coordination with the other muscles of the body.

- **<u>Stability Training to Avoid Injuries</u>**

Because stability training teaches the body to maintain control and stability during movements, even in erratic situations, it has a significant positive effect on preventing injuries. Proprioception, or the body's perception of movement, activity, and location, can be improved by activities that increase stability, such as single-leg exercises or the use of balancing boards. This increased awareness and control, by training the body to respond to abrupt changes in direction or surroundings, can significantly lower the chance of injury in daily activities as well as sporting undertakings.

- **Including Essential Duties in Your Everyday Schedule**

Without the need for regimented exercises, including core-strengthening activities into daily routines can make a substantial contribution to the development of core strength. Continuous and practical core training may be obtained by engaging in activities like sitting with an engaged and upright posture, utilizing the stairs, and engaging mindfully in core-involved tasks like cleaning or gardening. Furthermore, including low-impact exercises like yoga or Pilates in everyday life might help to further improve core stability and strength.

- **Hard Core Workouts to Get the Best Strength**

Complex sports, along with entire body motions, resistance, and difficult postures, can be pretty effective for folks who want to reach the finest stages of core energy. Exercises like Turkish get-ups, which integrate motion, electricity, and balance, or the pall of presses, which prevent rotation and increase middle persistence, are examples of this type of workout. Hanging leg raises additionally work the whole anterior chain of the middle. These complicated exercises educate the middle to function in unison with the rest of the body, matching the needs of everyday living and athletic overall performance further to strengthening the center.

The intention of strengthening the middle is to create a foundation of stability and strength that pervades every pass, as opposed to just getting 6%. The fundamental, stabilizing, and supporting roles of the core in total power practice apply

To movements in all planes. Exercises ranging from fundamental planks to difficult movements may be utilized to broaden this middle ground. Stability schooling is an essential part of any health software because it has the greater benefit of preventing injuries. Including middle sports in everyday sports guarantees that those important muscle tissues are continuously used and evolved. Last but not least, complicated workouts placed the middle through loads of challenges, leading to top energy and stability that improve each day's activities and sports performance.

CHAPTER 8
OLYMPIC LIFTING AND POWERLIFTING

- ## <u>Powerlifting Overview</u>

Powerlifting stands out within the international of electricity sports as it concentrates simplest on achieving maximum power in 3 lifts: the squat, bench press, and deadlift. A wonderful deal of effort is made to improve the method, power, and general capacity of those three motions through practitioners. In comparison to Olympic lifting, which emphasizes energy and approach, or bodybuilding, which prioritizes seems, powerlifting is largely focused on the whole weight lifted during competition.

- ## <u>Olympic Lifting: A Synopsis of the Equipment</u>

Athletes participating in Olympic lifting, sometimes referred to as weightlifting, must do two lifts: the snatch and the clean and jerk. It is a dynamic sport. These are intricate actions that call for not just physical strength but also explosive force, dexterity, and exact technique. In a snatch, the barbell is raised from the floor to above in a single action, whereas in a clean and jerk, the weight is pulled to the shoulders and then thrown aloft in two stages.

- ## <u>Power Training's Foundational Ideas and Methods</u>

Olympic lifting and powerlifting are both based on power training. It is based on the idea of overload, which is raising the weight gradually to put strain on the muscles and promote growth. Periodized training, which divides exercises into cycles of increasing intensity, is essential to both sports. Additionally, complex exercises that work many muscle groups at once are emphasized in power training, giving an all-encompassing foundation of strength.

- ## <u>Including Strength Training Activities in a Program for Bodybuilding</u>

A bodybuilding plan can benefit significantly from using Olympic lifting and powerlifting power education activities. These workout routines boost muscular growth and uncooked strength, giving bodybuilders a sturdy basis on which to create their physiques. Exercises like squats and deadlifts are already not unusual in bodybuilding due to how well they increase the bulk in the legs and lower back, respectively. Olympic lifts' explosiveness can also help to bolster the neuromuscular hyperlink that is vital for muscle boom and coordination.

- ## <u>8.5 Heavy Lifting Safety and Equipment</u>

Safety must be prioritized when performing heavy lifting, such as powerlifting and Olympic lifting, as a way to prevent accidents. To shop their spine and joints, athletes want to master secure lifting practices. They often use supportive, stable footwear, knee sleeves, wrist wraps, belts, and different safety tools. These sports activities' particular gyms have platforms, pinnacle-notch barbells, bumper plates, and racks made to face up to the heavy weights utilized in exercise and competition.

Both Olympic lifting and powerlifting are outstanding features within the international sport of strength athletics. Through the use of their own methods, beliefs, and schooling regimens, they each exceed the constraints of human electricity. These sports provide bodybuilders with a wealth of strategies to enhance their personal exercises, increasing their power and appearance. However, the full-size weights these athletes raise necessitate strict adherence to protection processes and device utilization, guaranteeing that their quest for strength does not come at the price of their health. Athletes that compete in powerlifting and Olympic lifting represent the highest level of energy through rigorous schooling and preparation.

CHAPTER 9

BODYBUILDERS' CARDIOVASCULAR EXERCISE PROGRAM

- ## The Role of the Cardiovascular System in Muscle Growth

Cardiovascular exercise plays a complex and sometimes underappreciated function in muscle building. Cardiovascular exercise is important for bodybuilders not just for burning fat and increasing endurance but also for accelerating muscle recovery. Cardio helps move essential nutrients to the muscles and facilitates repair and development by boosting blood flow. An effective cardiovascular system can also enhance general metabolic health, which promotes an anabolic environment favorable to muscle growth.

- ## Cardio: Selecting Between Intense and Low: Shifting the Balance

The bodybuilding world is still debating between high- and low-intensity cardio. Because of its well-known capacity to burn fat without sacrificing muscle, low-intensity steady-state (LISS) cardio is a mainstay of many bodybuilders' regimens. Conversely, high-intensity interval training (HIIT) has become more popular due to its effectiveness and capacity to dramatically increase metabolism. Effective integration of cardio requires striking a balance between time and intensity to support muscle growth objectives and reduce muscle catabolism.

- ## Using Interval Training to Reduce Fat and Maintain Muscle

One effective tactic for bodybuilders looking to reduce body fat and maintain muscular mass is interval training. Bodybuilders may create a significant calorie burn and trigger a positive hormonal response that supports muscle maintenance by alternating periods of high-intensity work with rest or low-intensity activity. Interval training may also be tailored to other modalities, including jogging, cycling, or rowing, giving cardiovascular exercises more variation and focus.

- ## Cardiovascular Well-Being: A Lifelong Dedication

Cardiovascular health is a lifetime commitment for bodybuilders, rather than just a means to an end. Maintaining a healthy heart and circulatory system is a more important goal than aiming for an attractive body. Frequent aerobic activity lowers the chance of developing heart disease, high blood pressure, and other illnesses. Bodybuilders guarantee they are developing a foundation for long-term health in addition to muscle by dedicating themselves to a regimen that incorporates cardio.

Cardiovascular Health and Strength Training in Harmony

For bodybuilders, striking a balance between power education and cardiovascular fitness is vital. Although growing muscular mass is regularly the main objective, ignoring the coronary heart might have bad outcomes for overall performance and fitness. Cardio has to be blanketed into programming in a way that enhances resistance schooling and body composition, maintaining a strong cardiovascular machine without sacrificing muscular advantage. Bodybuilders might also create a comprehensive approach that nourishes their bodies on the inside and out by seeing cardiovascular pastime as a supplement to electricity education in preference to as a substitute.

Basically, cardiovascular conditioning goes much beyond the straightforward goal of burning calories when it comes to bodybuilding. It is a complex part of an all-encompassing training program that promotes muscular growth, facilitates recuperation, and maintains general health. Cardio may be a powerful ally when used wisely, working in tandem with strength training to develop a strong, resilient, and well-rounded athlete. Cardio guarantees that the bodybuilder's heart is as strong as their physique, whether through steady-state workouts or the dynamic bursts of interval training. This creates a synergy between endurance and strength for a lifetime of fitness and well-being.

CHAPTER 10
STRATEGIES FOR LONG–TERM SUCCESS

- ### Creating and Upholding Goals

Setting unique desires is the first step in developing a long-term bodybuilding plan. These dreams need to cross past superficial appearances or transient victories to include lengthy-term well-being, slow strength growth, and higher overall performance. It is crucial to often reflect and be bendy as a way to uphold those dreams. A practitioner wishes to be on defense and prepared to modify their goals in response to the ups and downs of life, changes in their bodies, and growing private obligations.

- ### Overcoming Difficulties and Failures

A necessary companion on the path to bodybuilding dominance is adversity. Such obstacles must be overcome with resiliency and a strategic mentality. Any kind of setback—injuries, plateaus, or personal struggles—must be tackled from a solution-focused perspective. It is essential to develop a mental toolkit that includes persistence, patience, and problem-solving skills. Every challenge overcome strengthens mental toughness and creates an unbreakable spirit, both of which are essential for continuous advancement.

- ## <u>The Psychological Effects of Bodybuilding</u>

Bodybuilding may have a range of psychological impacts, from the powerful surge of endorphins to the intimidating threat of burnout. It is crucial to acknowledge the psychological and emotional toll that constant training takes. In order to keep their psychological well-being intact, athletes need to practice mindfulness, get enough sleep, and enjoy life outside of the gym. This self-awareness makes sure that the goal of building stronger muscles also builds stronger mental toughness.

- ## <u>Companionship, Competition, and Amity</u>

In the ring of iron and perspiration, friendships frequently flourish. Training partners turn into confidants; rivals provide motivation for development; and friendships arise out of the fabric of shared adversity. This fellowship is a powerful source of encouragement, responsibility, and support. Friendships act as a safety net in case one falters, while rivalries push one to new heights. The group experience adds value to the individual search, creating a fabric of common experiences that strengthen one's commitment.

- ## <u>Maintaining and Increasing Muscle Throughout Life</u>

The brief glory of winning an opposition or the momentary victory of reaching a non-public quality elevate no longer constitute the middle of bodybuilding. The real triumph is found in the pursuit of lifetime health—muscle increase and cautious maintenance during the years. This necessitates a well-rounded approach to restoration, weight-reduction plan, and workout with an emphasis on lengthy-term behaviors that assist energy and health. It is essential to be aware of the body's transferring necessities and to adjust methods accordingly so that the golden years aren't a sign of a weak spot but rather an alternative to a nicely-stored temple of muscle.

Stepping onto the road to long-term bodybuilding fulfillment entails stepping into an adventure of self-transformation that goes beyond the physical. It is a hard adventure that requires an aggregate of strength of will, making plans, and a steadfast willpower to self-develop. Through this furnace of labor and perspiration, one develops a sturdy frame and a hard spirit, which might be ready to face life's ups and downs. The gym becomes a little model of the real world, wherein people establish and attain goals, triumph over demanding situations, and sharpen and test their spirits. The bodybuilder discovers the key additives of long-term achievement—power, intelligence, friendship, and the unwavering pursuit of a lifestyle lived at its physical peak—within the alchemy of iron and ambition.

MACRONUTRIENT BALANCE, CALORIE EXCESS, AND MEAL TIMING ALL PLAY A ROLE IN CREATING AN OPTIMAL MUSCLE–BUILDING DIET PLAN CHART.

BREAKFAST

- One cup of oats, topped with almonds and a banana, boiled in water or almond milk
- Three big eggs, prepared in whatever way you choose (boil, scramble, poach, etc.).
- Snack of one serving of whey protein shake made with water or a milk substitute
- a tablespoon of honey and a pinch of chia seeds drizzled over a cup of plain Greek yogurt
- One medium-sized apple, peeled and sliced
- 6 oz. of grilled or baked chicken breast
- One cup of cooked quinoa
- One cup of steamed or sautéed mixed vegetables in olive oil
- Snack Size: 1/2 an avocado, sliced
- One cup of fat-free cottage cheese
- 1/4 cup of mixed nuts before a workout
- Cooked brown rice equals a half cup.
- One medium-roasted sweet potato after exercise

- ➤ Protein Drink: Whey protein, diluted with water, 1 serving
- ➤ Banana = 1 Hearty Supper
- ➤ Grilled or baked salmon (around 6 ounces)
- ➤ Steamed broccoli, one cup
- ➤ Various leafy vegetables Two cups of salad with a dressing of olive oil and vinegar

SNACK TIME (IF NEEDED)

One serving of casein protein powder blended with water.

Important Considerations:

- Maintaining adequate hydration throughout the day is essential; try to drink 8 glasses of water.
- Your demands, degree of exercise, and desire to gain muscle mass should inform how much and how often you eat.
- Include protein, complex carbs, and healthy fats at each of your three main meals a day.
- Your workout routine may inform the timing of your meals, giving you the fuel you need to get through your workout and the nutrients you need to recuperate.
- Consult with a nutritionist or dietitian for a tailored plan, especially if you have dietary limitations or other health problems.
- This diet plan is flexible and may be adjusted to meet the specific food choices, intolerances, and dietary requirements of each individual. It's a

general outline that emphasizes eating a variety of nutritious foods to aid in muscle building.

Summary

"Men who want to grow muscle do well to mix intense exercise with well-planned meals. Muscle size and strength may be increased by resistance training because it repairs damaged muscle fibers as you sleep. It's a methodical path that combines effort with rest and requires perseverance, tolerance, and discipline. The dedication it takes to build a stronger self is mirrored in the physical changes that occur with regular exercise".